FAST
YOUR WAY OUT

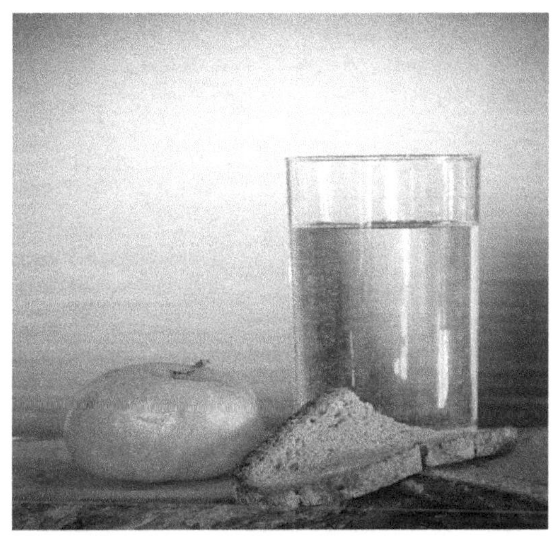

A Complete Expert's Guide For Hormonal Balance, Menstrual Health, and Weight Control for Women Through Fasting

Thelma Pauley

TABLE CONTENT

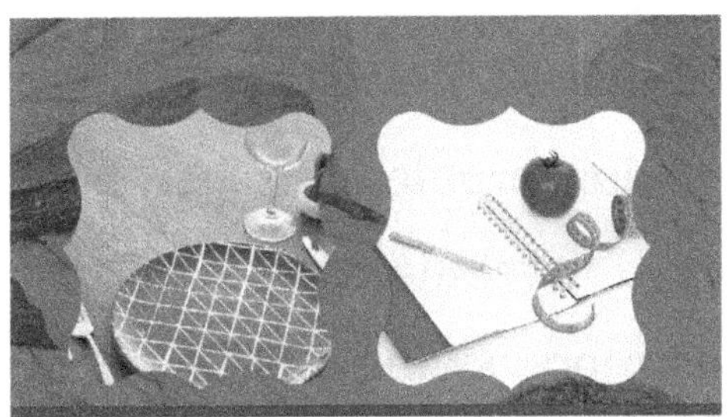

FAST YOUR WAY OUT

*A Complete Expert's Guide For Hormonal Balance,
Menstrual Health, and Weight Control for Women
Through Fasting*

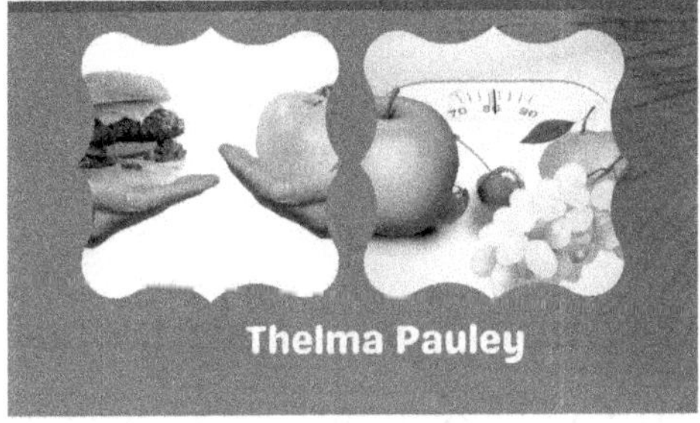

Thelma Pauley

Introduction

Sarah had one major problem in her busy life: hormonal irregularities. These imbalances caused mood swings, fatigue, and weight gain related to her menstrual cycle. Sarah has tried all she could by going to doctors and health professionals, but her quest for balance was always just out of reach.

Sarah was reading through social media one day and saw a picture of someone she already knew, Emily. Emily was young and confident. Sarah was impressed by Emily's transformation and realized that fasting, as prescribed in the book "Fast Your Way Out," was the secret to her transformation.

Sarah's optimism grew as Emily described her approach to treating hormonal abnormalities and finding balance through fasting. She concluded that fasting could be the missing link in its overall well-being.

Many women including Sarah herself have found it very hard to balance work, family, and their personal lives. Hormonal imbalances, including mood swings, irregular sleep patterns, and weight issues are a serious problem.

Despite attempting various approaches, discovering the correct balance can prove challenging. Then there are pivotal moments, such as the experience of a friend like Emily, who derived empowerment through fasting with the guidance of "Fast Your Way Out."

This book will serve as a resource for women facing specific health challenges. It covers the science of fasting, techniques for balancing hormones, and the art of weight management. You will learn about hormone-focused eating and how to successfully end a fast.

Women will discover how fasting can empower them to regain control of their health as we go through this book. It lays out pathways to unleash energy, leading to a state of well-being and an unstoppable self.

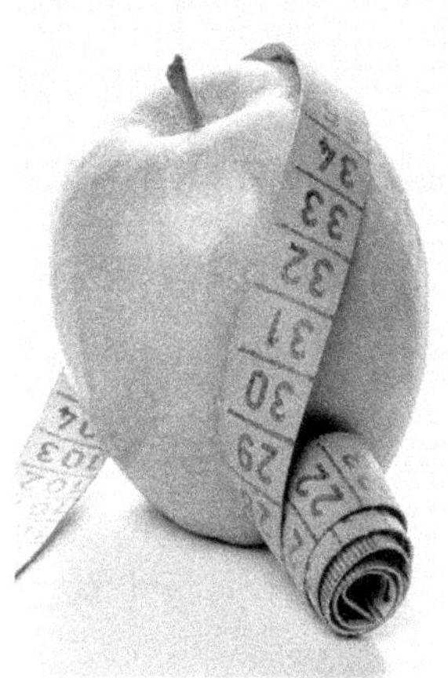

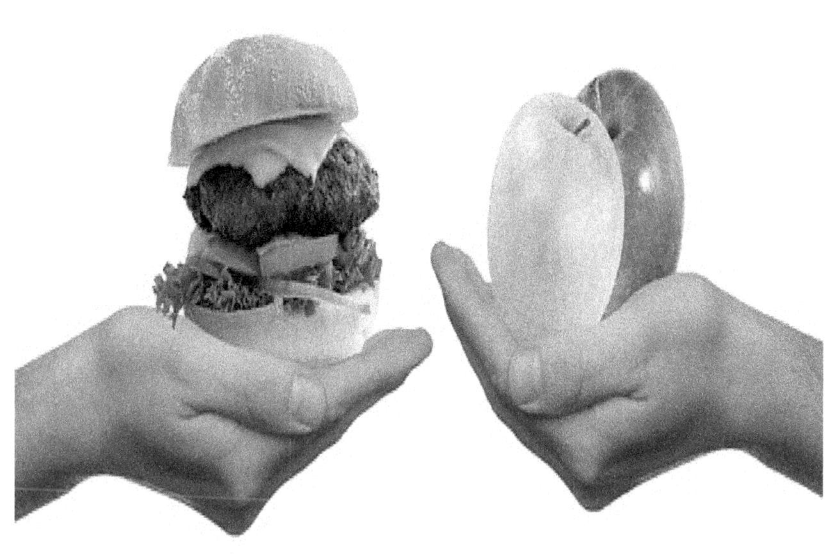

Chapter 1: Understanding Hormones

Hormones are the quiet conductors in the delicate dance of life within the human body, coordinating a symphony of biological events. This chapter acts as a compass for us, guiding us through the complex relationships between hormones, and helping us to comprehend their enormous effects on women's health and well-being.

The Hormonal Balance: The Harmony of A Woman's Health

Think of your hormones as individual instruments in a well-tuned orchestra, each one adding to the overall symphony of life. Hormones are the composers that shape your health story, from the heart's rhythmic beats to the menstrual cycle's complex dance.

To put it simply, hormones are messengers that the body produces through different glands. They provide messages to organs and tissues via the bloodstream, affecting everything from mood to metabolism.

The Vital Hormones Affecting Women's Health

Hormones are the quiet conductors in the intricate world of women's health, arranging a complex symphony. Maintaining equilibrium and overall health is largely dependent on these messengers, which are involved in reproductive cycles and metabolic functions. Now let's explore the key hormones that have a big impact on women's health:

1. Estrogen

Many people believe that estrogen is the main hormone in women. It promotes reproductive health, controls the menstrual cycle, and helps to preserve bone density.

Menstrual Cycle: During the first half of the menstrual cycle, estrogen levels rise, encouraging the uterine lining to grow in preparation for pregnancy.

Healthy Reproduction: Beyond the menstrual cycle, estrogen affects the health of the ovaries, eggs, and reproductive system as a whole, all of which are important components of fertility.

Bone Health: For bone density to be maintained, estrogen is essential. Bone loss can result from decreased estrogen levels, particularly during menopause.

2. Progesterone

In addition to working in tandem with estrogen to control the menstrual cycle, progesterone is essential for both pregnancy and good reproductive health in general.

Periodic phase:

Progesterone levels rise in the second part of the menstrual cycle, preparing the uterine lining for a possible pregnancy and assisting in the event of an early pregnancy.

Pregnancy Support:

By protecting the lining of the uterus and averting potentially miscarriage-causing contractions, progesterone aids in the maintenance of a pregnancy.

Endocrine Balance:

It functions as an estrogen counterweight, promoting hormonal balance and halting the uterine lining's overgrowth.

3. Testosterone

Testosterone, which is frequently linked to men, is also found in women and affects their vitality, muscular mass, and reproductive health.

Power and Vitality: Testosterone plays a role in maintaining a healthy body composition, muscle strength, and general energy levels.

Appetite:

It affects arousal and sexual desire. Women who have balanced libidos have higher levels of testosterone in their bodies.

System of Reproduction:

Testosterone supports healthy reproductive systems overall and is implicated in ovarian function.

4. Insulin

Insulin is a vital component of metabolic health, not just for women, but especially for those who suffer from disorders like polycystic ovarian syndrome (PCOS).

Rules for Blood Sugar:

Insulin promotes the uptake of glucose into cells for energy, which helps control blood sugar levels.

Connection with PCOS:

Women with PCOS frequently have insulin resistance, which exacerbates hormonal imbalances and metabolic problems.

5. Cortisol

The hormone cortisol, which is frequently linked to stress, is essential for the body's reaction to different types of stress.

Reaction to Stress:

In reaction to stress, cortisol aids in the mobilization of energy reserves, readying the body for the "fight or flight" reaction.

The Immune System:

It affects the immune system and aids in controlling immunological reactions and inflammation.

Routine Pace:

Cortisol affects energy levels and sleep habits, with a natural daily rhythm of spiking in the early morning and declining during the day.

6. Thyroid Hormones

The entire energy balance and metabolism are regulated by thyroid hormones, particularly T3 and T4.

The abdomen:

Thyroid hormones affect the body's general metabolic function by influencing the rate at which food is converted into energy.

Temperature of Body:

They help to keep the balance of other hormones and aid in the control of body temperature.

Effect on Pelvic Health:

Thyroid dysfunction emphasizes the interdependence of hormones by influencing menstrual regularity and fertility.

Gaining an understanding of the complex relationship between these hormones is essential for managing women's health.

A variety of health problems, including irregular menstruation and metabolic diseases, can be attributed to imbalances in these hormonal players. The secret is to keep everything in balance.

Diet, exercise, and stress reduction are important lifestyle choices that promote hormonal equilibrium. As we delve deeper into our investigation, we'll see how fasting can function as a transforming tool to support the health of these vital hormones.

Hormones' Effect on Your Well-Being

Knowing the symphony of hormones helps us recognize how imbalances can throw off the harmony of health. Because hormones are interrelated, changes in one can have an impact on the balance of the other hormones:

Healthy Menstruation and Hormones

The menstrual cycle is regulated by the subtle interactions between progesterone and estrogen. Period irregularities, PMS symptoms, and more serious illnesses like polycystic ovarian syndrome (PCOS) can all be caused by imbalances.

Weight Control and Hormones

The thyroid hormone, cortisol, and insulin work together in the body's metabolic dance. Errors in this dance routine may lead to weight gain or make it difficult to lose excess weight.

Emotional Health and Hormones

Hormones have an emotional influence in addition to their physical effects. We can better manage stress, mood swings, and the complex relationship between hormonal and mental health when we are aware of this connection.

Establishing the Groundwork for Your Fasting Adventure

As we come to the end of this first chapter, think of it as the base from which we will expand our knowledge. Deciphering the hormonal symphony is the first step toward weight control, menstrual health, and hormone balance.

We'll look at how fasting becomes the empowering conductor in the upcoming chapters, balancing these essential components for your overall healt

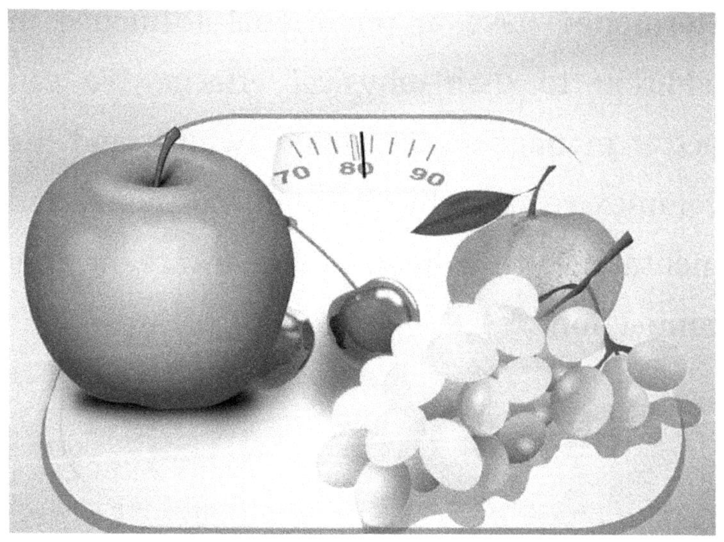

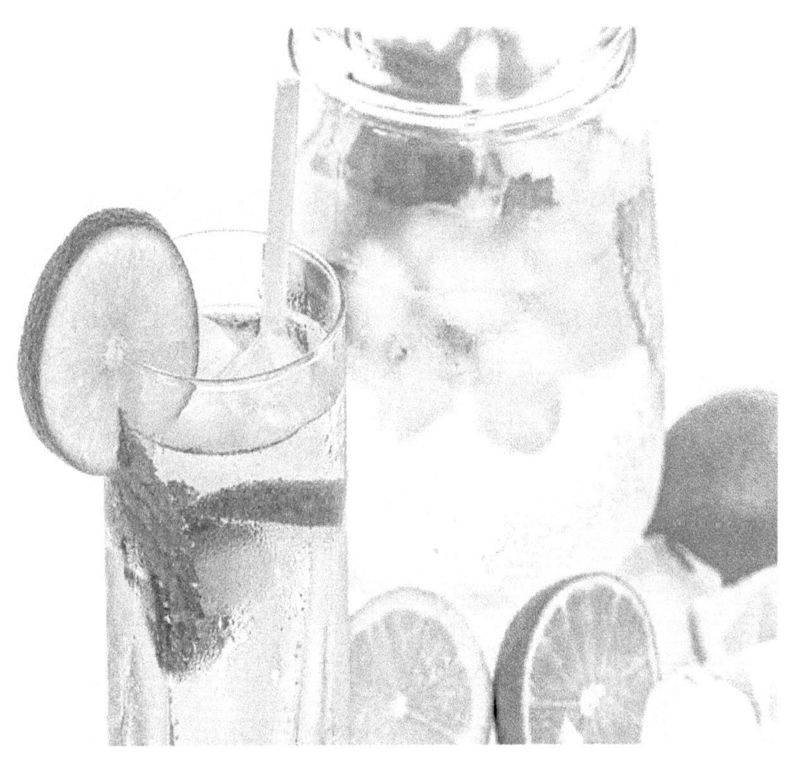

Chapter 2: The Art of Fasting

Fasting, often surrounded by myths and misconceptions, can be demystified by understanding its principles and exploring various approaches. In this chapter, we will delve into the basics of fasting, different fasting methods, and how fasting influences hormones, menstrual health, and weight control. Additionally, we'll discuss how to lay the groundwork for a successful fasting journey.

Fasting Demystified

Fasting is not just about abstaining from food; it's a deliberate choice with potential health benefits. Demystifying fasting involves understanding its essence – a period of intentional abstention from eating. This practice has been embraced for centuries across cultures, not solely as a religious or spiritual observance but also for its impact on health.

Fasting is not synonymous with starvation; it is a controlled and purposeful approach to give the body a break from constant digestion, allowing it to focus on repair and rejuvenation. During fasting, the body shifts from using glucose as a primary energy source to burning stored fats, a process known as ketosis.

Different Methods for Fasting

Fasting is a flexible practice that may be tailored to fit different lifestyles, interests, and health objectives. Every technique provides a different viewpoint on when and how to fast, enabling people to select a fasting schedule that suits their requirements.

Here are a few well-known methods for fasting:

1. Improved Intermittent Fasting:

16/8 Method:

This method entails a 16-hour fast every day, followed by an 8-hour eating window. For instance, a person might eat from 12:00 pm to 8:00 pm and then fast from 8:00 pm to 12:00 pm the next day.

14/10 Method: This strategy reduces the fasting window to 14 hours with a 10-hour feeding window, much like the 16/8 method.

2. Other Day Fasting

Revised Other Day Fasting:

With this strategy, you can consume up to 25–25% of your usual calories on fasting days. On days when they are not fasting, people are able to eat.

Entire Day-by-Day Fasting:

In this more stringent version, people only consume calories once every other day.

3. A 24-Hour Fast

Consume, Stop, Consume:

This regimen calls for one or two 24-hour fasts every week. For example, someone may have dinner at 7:00 p.m. and skip breakfast the next day at 7:00 p.m.

Diet of Warriors:

This strategy is eating one big meal at night within a 4-hour eating window and taking little amounts of raw fruits and vegetables during the day.

4. 48-Hour Fasting

Extended Fasting:

Extended fasting is a 48-hour period during which no food is consumed. You might use this strategy once or twice a month.

The 5:2 Diet

People eat five days a week at regular intervals and only take in 500–600 calories on the two non-consecutive days.

5. Limited Eating Time

Initial Time-Restricted Feeding:
This approach entails a period of fasting after eating solely in the morning, say from 6:00 am to 2:00 pm.

Restricted Feeding Due to Late Times:
On the other hand, people can eat from 12:00 pm to 8:00 pm while continuing their fast into the morning.

6. Unplanned Meal Skipping

This adaptable strategy entails ignoring meals when you're not hungry and paying attention to your body's hunger signals. It permits intuitive feeding and is not restricted to any certain timetable.

Evaluations

Customization:

The degree to which a fasting method works for each person differs. The best approach is determined in part by individual criteria like age, gender, health, and lifestyle.

Aqueous:

Regardless of how you choose to fast, it's important to stay hydrated. Black coffee, herbal teas, and water are typically permitted during fasting times.

High-Nutrient Foods:

To make sure the body gets the vitamins and minerals it needs, it's critical to concentrate on nutrient-dense, whole meals during eating windows.

Selecting the appropriate fasting strategy requires taking into account lifestyle choices, medical issues, and personal preferences. Before starting any kind of fasting routine, it is best to speak with medical authorities, especially if you have any underlying medical concerns. Positive experiences with fasting are also enhanced by gradual implementation and regular hydration.

How Fasting Affects Hormones, Menstrual Health, and Weight Control

1. Hormones:

Regulation of Insulin:

Insulin, a hormone that controls blood sugar levels, can be better regulated by fasting. Fasting has been shown to improve weight control and reduce the risk of type 2 diabetes by lowering insulin resistance.

Increase in Growth Hormones: Growth hormone production is increased during fasting, which may aid in fat loss and muscle preservation.

Release of Norepinephrine:

The hormone norepinephrine, which aids in the body's breakdown of fat for energy, is released when fasting is undertaken.

2. Menstrual Health

Impact on the Menstrual Cycle:

For some women, fasting—especially intermittent fasting—may have an impact on their menstrual periods. It's critical to take into account unique reactions from each person and think about customized fasting strategies.

Endocrine Balance:

There are differences in how fasting affects hormonal balance, and women should be aware of how it affects their menstrual health.

3. Management of Weight **Adaptability to Metabolism:**

By promoting metabolic flexibility, fasting enables the body to utilize fat reserves and glucose as fuel. This could help in managing weight effectively.

Restrictions on Calorie:

Although fasting can lead to calorie restriction, there are other advantages of fasting besides calorie reduction. The hormonal and metabolic systems involved in weight regulation are impacted by fasting.

A Holistic Perspective:

Fasting for weight loss often works best when accompanied with a holistic strategy that takes into account factors like mindful eating, regular exercise, and general well-being.

To put it simply, fasting has beneficial effects on weight control, menstrual health, and hormone balancing. It promotes metabolic flexibility, increases hormones that aid in fat reduction, and aids in insulin regulation.

Individual responses, however, differ, particularly when it comes to menstruation health, underscoring the necessity of tailored strategies. A complete lifestyle approach combined with fasting increases its efficacy in managing weight.

Setting the Foundation for Your Fasting Journey

Embarking on a fasting journey requires thoughtful preparation. Setting the foundation involves understanding personal health conditions, consulting healthcare professionals if necessary, and gradually easing into fasting routines. Hydration, nutrient-dense meals during eating windows, and mindful food choices are crucial components.

Establishing realistic goals is paramount. Whether aiming for weight loss, improved energy levels, or overall well-being, defining clear objectives helps track progress and stay motivated.

Additionally, recognizing the individual nature of fasting experiences promotes self-compassion and flexibility in adapting fasting practices to evolving needs.

In conclusion, the art of fasting encompasses more than abstaining from food; it involves a nuanced understanding of its principles and a personalized approach.

By demystifying fasting, exploring diverse methods, acknowledging hormonal influences, and laying a solid foundation, individuals can embark on a fasting journey that aligns with their well-being goals.

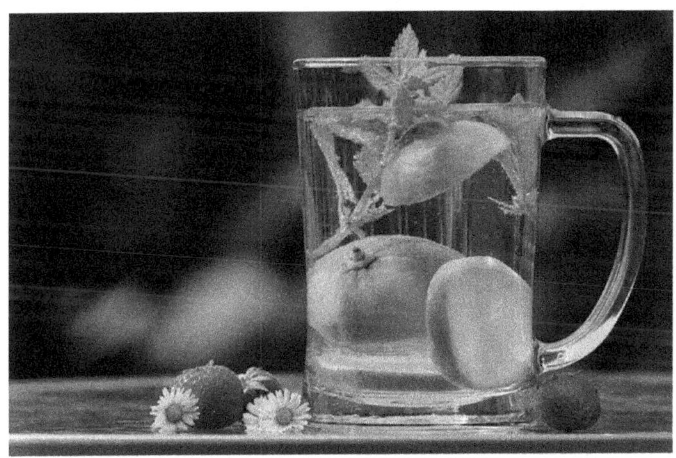

Chapter 3: Menstrual Health Unveiled

We will explore the complexities of the menstrual cycle, learn how fasting can be a supportive ally in promoting menstrual well-being, and address common issues that many people encounter during this normal biological process as we unravel the mysteries surrounding menstrual health in this chapter.

Understanding the Menstrual Cycle

The female body goes through an intriguing and intricate journey during the menstrual cycle. It consists of a sequence of hormonal changes that prime the uterus for a possible pregnancy and lasts for around 28 days. Gaining an appreciation of this cycle is essential to understanding the delicate hormone balance involved.

Menstrual Phase:

The uterine lining sheds during menstruation, which marks the start of the cycle.

Follicular Phase:

The uterine lining thickens and hormones cause the ovaries to create an egg.

Ovulation:

The midpoint of the cycle is marked by the release of an egg from the ovary.

Luteal Phase:

The body gets ready for pregnancy; the cycle resumes if conception is unsuccessful.

Menstrual health can be supported by fasting when it is done mindfully and sensitively. It's crucial to remember that everyone reacts differently to fasting, so any alterations should be carefully considered.

How Fasting May Affect Menstrual Health

Insulin Sensitivity: Insulin sensitivity can be improved by fasting, which may help to improve hormonal balance during the menstrual cycle.

Reduction of Inflammation:

Some types of fasting have the potential to lower inflammation, which is advantageous for people who are uncomfortable during their periods.

Endocrine Balance:

Fasting may have an impact on menstruation regularity by balancing hormones generally.

Menstrual Health and Fasting Considerations

Customized Method:

Since each person is different, what works for one might not work for another. It's critical to take a customized approach to fasting, taking into account each person's unique health circumstances and reactions.

Nutrition and Hydration:

It's crucial to maintain adequate hydration and nourishment at mealtimes. Menstrual health can be impacted by nutritional deficits and dehydration.

Warm Salutations:

If you're thinking about fasting, introduce it gradually and gently so the body can adjust without suffering unnecessary stress.

Dealing with Typical Menstrual Issues

Menstrual difficulties are widespread, and although fasting may have some advantages, it's important to deal with these difficulties thoroughly.

Typical Menstrual Problems and Solutions

Pain and Discomfort:

Warm compresses, light exercise, and staying hydrated can all help relieve period cramps in addition to fasting.

Anomalous Cycles:

If fasting interferes with menstruation regularity, it might be helpful to modify the fasting window or look into other options.

Psychological Health:

Emotional wellness is just as important to menstrual health as physical health. It's essential to engage in self-care and get emotional assistance.

Diet:

For menstrual health, a diet rich in nutrients and well-balanced is essential. Overall nutrition shouldn't be compromised by fasting.

The Mind-Body Link:

It is essential to understand the mind-body link. Getting enough sleep and managing stress are important for overall menstrual health.

In conclusion, a comprehensive view of women's well-being can be achieved by comprehending the menstrual cycle, recognizing the possible effects of fasting on menstrual health, and tackling prevalent issues.

It highlights that for a balanced and healthy menstrual experience, a customized approach, careful awareness of body signals, and the integration of holistic practices are necessary.

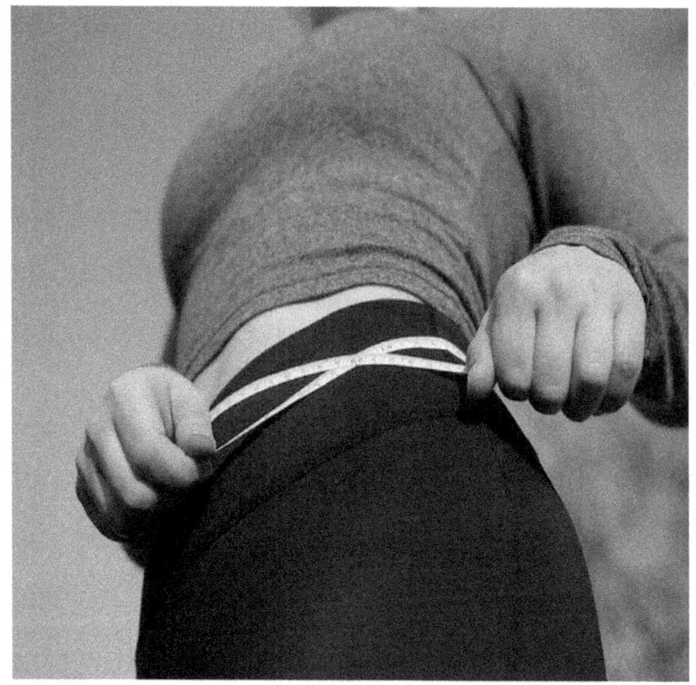

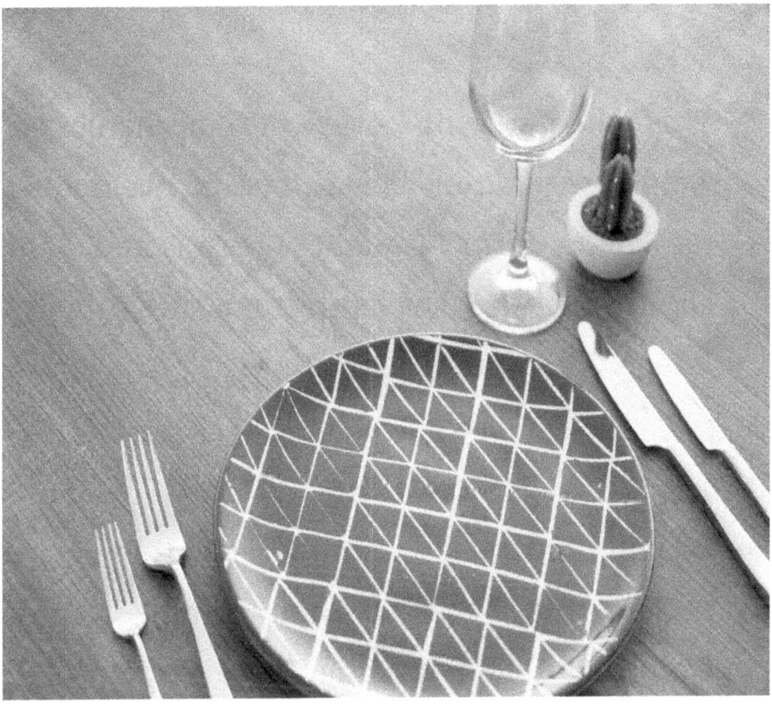

Chapter 4: Expert Guidance on Weight Control

This chapter will cover the mechanics of weight regulation, doable fasting techniques for long-term weight loss, and the significance of developing a positive body-image. Allow me to explain it simply.

Dynamics of Weight Control

Weight control is a nuanced interplay of factors that goes beyond simple calorie counting. Understanding these dynamics is essential for adopting effective and sustainable strategies for managing weight. Let's delve into the key components that shape the dynamics of weight control:

1. Caloric Balance:

Calories In vs. Calories Out:

Weight control fundamentally revolves around the balance between the calories consumed through food and beverages and the calories expended through metabolic processes and physical activity.

Energy Surplus and Deficit:

Consuming more calories than the body needs leads to weight gain, while a caloric deficit, where fewer calories are consumed than expended, results in weight loss.

2. Metabolic Rate

Basal Metabolic Rate (BMR):

This represents the number of calories the body needs at rest to maintain basic physiological functions. Factors such as age, gender, genetics, and muscle mass influence BMR.

Metabolic Flexibility:

Fasting and certain dietary practices can impact metabolic flexibility, allowing the body to efficiently switch between using glucose and stored fats for energy.

3. Nutrient Intake

Quality of Calories:

It's not just about the quantity of calories but also the quality of the nutrients. Nutrient-dense foods provide essential vitamins, minerals, and other compounds that support overall health.

Balanced Nutrition:

A well-balanced diet ensures that the body receives the necessary nutrients for optimal function, contributing to overall well-being during weight management.

4. Hormonal Influences

Insulin:

Regulates blood sugar levels and plays a crucial role in fat storage. Insulin sensitivity, influenced by factors including diet and fasting, affects weight control.

Ghrelin and Leptin:

These hormones regulate hunger and satiety. Fasting can influence their levels, impacting appetite and eating behaviors.

5. Psychological Factors

Emotional Eating:
Psychological factors such as stress, boredom, or emotions can influence eating habits. Building awareness of emotional triggers is crucial for sustainable weight control.

Mindful Eating:
Cultivating mindfulness around food choices, savoring each bite, and paying attention to hunger and fullness cues contribute to a healthier relationship with food.

Exercise and Caloric Expenditure:

Regular physical activity contributes to weight control by burning calories and improving overall metabolic health.

Strength Training:

Building and maintaining muscle mass through strength training can positively impact metabolism and support weight management.

Understanding the dynamics of weight control involves recognizing the multifaceted nature of the body's response to various inputs, including food, activity, and psychological factors.

Adopting a holistic approach that considers these dynamics is key to developing effective and sustainable strategies for achieving and maintaining a healthy weight.

Methods of Fasting for Long-Term Weight Loss

Fasting is more than just a band-aid treatment; it's not a one-size-fits-all approach. Embarking on a journey of long-term weight loss requires sustainable and effective methods.

Fasting can be a powerful tool in this endeavor, promoting fat loss, metabolic health, and overall well-being. Using fasting techniques that fit your objectives and lifestyle is essential to sustainable weight management.

Here are several methods of fasting that have shown promise for long-term weight loss:

1. Intermittent Fasting (IF):

16/8 Method: Involves a daily fasting period of 16 hours, followed by an 8-hour eating window. This method is adaptable to various lifestyles and can be sustained long-term.

5:2 Diet: Incorporates two non-consecutive days of very low-calorie intake (around 500-600 calories) and regular eating on the other five days. This method provides flexibility and can be sustainable over the long term.

2. Alternate-Day Fasting

Modified Approach: Allows for a reduced calorie intake (20-25% of normal) on fasting days rather than complete abstinence. This modification can make alternate-day fasting more sustainable.

Complete Fasting:

Involves alternating between days of normal eating and days of complete fasting. While effective, adherence over the long term may be challenging for some individuals.

3. Extended Fasting

24-Hour Fasting:

This method involves fasting for a complete 24-hour period once or twice a week. It can be practiced intermittently for long-term weight management.

48-Hour Fasting:

Longer fasting periods may provide deeper metabolic benefits. However, they require careful consideration and may not be suitable for everyone.

4. Time-Restricted Eating

Early Time-Restricted Feeding: Limits eating to the early part of the day, such as a 6:00 am to 2:00 pm window. This aligns with the body's natural circadian rhythms and may be sustainable in the long term.

Late Time-Restricted Feeding: Involves eating between 12:00 pm and 8:00 pm, with fasting hours extending into the morning. This approach is adaptable and can be maintained over the long term.

5. Continuous Energy Restriction

Reduced-Calorie Diets:

While not fasting per se, adopting a continuous energy restriction by consuming fewer calories than the body expends can lead to gradual, sustainable weight loss over the long term.

6. Combination Approaches

Cyclic Fasting:

Alternating between periods of fasting and regular eating on a cyclic basis. This approach provides flexibility and may be more sustainable than strict, continuous fasting.

Fasting-Mimicking Diet:

Involves consuming a specific low-calorie and low-protein diet for a set number of days, mimicking the effects of fasting. This approach may be more palatable for long-term adherence.

Considerations for Long-Term Fasting

Personal Variability:

The effectiveness of fasting methods varies among individuals. It's essential to choose an approach that aligns with personal preferences, health conditions, and lifestyle.

Nutrient-Dense Eating:

Even during eating windows, focusing on nutrient-dense foods supports overall health and ensures that the body receives essential vitamins and minerals.

Regular Monitoring:

Regular check-ins with healthcare professionals can provide guidance and ensure that fasting practices align with individual health goals.

Mindful Consumption:

Eating isn't the only aspect of fasting; there are other aspects as well. A better relationship with food can be achieved by paying attention to your food choices, enjoying every meal, and learning to recognize your body's signals of hunger and fullness.

Gradual Introduction:

If you've never fasted before, go carefully. Increase the length of your fasts gradually so that your body can adjust to it.

Water:

Drink plenty of water when fasting. Black coffee, herbal teas, and water are all wise options. Sometimes, dehydration is confused with hunger.

Developing a Positive Connection with Your Body

Managing your weight is not simply a physical endeavor; it is intricately linked to your mental and emotional health as well. Developing a positive relationship with your body is essential to long-term weight control.

Means to Promote a Positive Body Image

Self-Compassion:

Treat oneself with kindness. Recognize that controlling your weight is a process and that your body is unique. Accept progress rather than perfection.

Body-Mind Link:

Pay attention to your body. Recognize its hunger and fullness cues. Become aware of your feelings toward various foods. Positive relationships can be powerfully fostered by the mind-body link.

Motivation:

Include any movement that makes you happy. Exercising is about appreciating what your body is capable of, not just about burning calories.

In summary, professional advice on managing weight entails comprehending the dynamics, implementing workable fasting techniques, and—above all—establishing a healthy rapport with your body. It's a comprehensive method that transcends scale measurements, emphasizing general wellbeing and appreciating the individuality of each person's path.

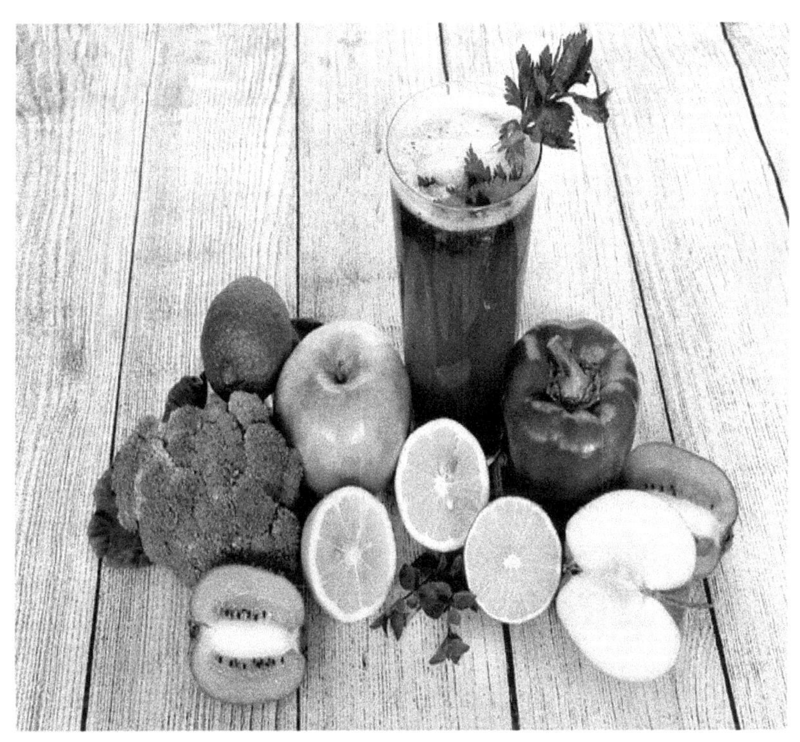

Chapter 5: Balancing Hormones through Expert Nutrition

This chapter will explain the role that nutrition plays in preserving hormonal balance, discuss foods that support hormonal harmony when fasting, and help you create a customized meal plan for ideal hormone balance. Now let's explore the realm of specialized nutrition for optimal hormonal balance.

The Role of Nutrition in Hormone Balance

Knowing how diet affects hormone balance is similar to learning your body's language. Food is a major factor in maintaining the complex hormonal dance that controls a range of physiological processes.

Fasting-Friendly Foods for Hormonal Balance

Selecting meals that support the fasting process is essential to navigating the fasting phase while preserving hormonal balance. These meals complement fasting objectives while also promoting general health.

1. Macronutrient Balance:

Proteins(Lean Proteins):

Incorporate foods such as tofu, lentils, and lean meats (fish, turkey and chicken)into your diet.

These lean proteins that help maintain muscle during periods of fasting. It are also required for the synthesis of hormones.

Fats: Good fats like nuts, seeds, avocado, and olive oil are essential for the synthesis of hormones and also give your body the necessary fats to help with satiety.

Complex carbohydrate:

Brown rice, quinoa, and sweet potatoes—these are carbs that release energy gradually aid in sustaining energy levels during fasting, prolonged energy and steady blood sugar levels, choose complex carbs like those found in whole grains and veggies.

2. Micronutrients

Vitamins:

Some vitamins, including vitamin D, are involved in the control of hormones. Vitamin D intake is influenced by fatty fish, fortified dairy products, and exposure to sunlight.

Minerals:

Hormone production involves minerals like zinc and magnesium. Leafy greens, nuts, and seeds should be included in your diet.

3. Foods High in Fiber:

These veggies, which are high in fiber and minerals, help you feel full. Consuming a lot of fiber promotes healthy digestion and helps control insulin levels. Good sources of fiber include whole grains, legumes, fruits, and vegetables.

4. Hydration:

Hormone transfer and general body processes depend on adequate hydration. Hydration can be achieved by the use of water, herbal teas, and fruit- and herb-infused water.

5. Avoiding Processed Foods:

Artificial additives and harmful fats, which can upset hormonal balance, are frequently found in processed foods. When possible, choose entire, unprocessed meals.

6.3 Creating a Diet Plan for Hormone Balancing

A diet plan that balances hormones and enhances fasting must carefully combine nutrient-dense foods with mindful eating techniques.

How to Create a Diet Plan for Hormone Balancing

1. Assess Your Nutritional Needs:

When assessing your nutritional needs, take into account variables such as age, gender, activity level, and health objectives.

2. Balanced Macronutrients:

Make sure that the proportions of proteins, lipids, and carbohydrates are all in balance at each meal. This promotes hormone synthesis and long-term energy production.

3. Incorporate entire Foods:

Give entire, high-nutrient foods precedence over processed alternatives. Your diet should be centered on whole grains, lean proteins, and fresh produce.

4. Mindful Eating Practices:

Recognize your body's signals of hunger and fullness. During meals, try to eat carefully, enjoy every bite, and stay away from distractions.

5. Hydration Routine:

Create a consistent schedule for staying hydrated. Strive to maintain a sufficient water intake throughout the day to support all body functions.

6. Adjust Based on Fasting Approach:

Modify your eating plan to work in tandem with the fasting strategy you've selected. Take into account the length of times you fast and modify your nutrient intake accordingly.

7. Continuous Observation and Modification:
Evaluate your body's reaction to the diet plan on a regular basis. Be willing to make changes when your nutritional demands and general health change.

In summary, skilled nutrition for hormonal balance entails a comprehensive strategy that takes into account mindful eating habits in addition to food composition.

Creating a nutrition plan around your fasting objectives benefits general health and well–being in addition to hormonal balance. Recall that on your path to ideal hormonal balance, it matters not only what you consume but also how you nourish your body.

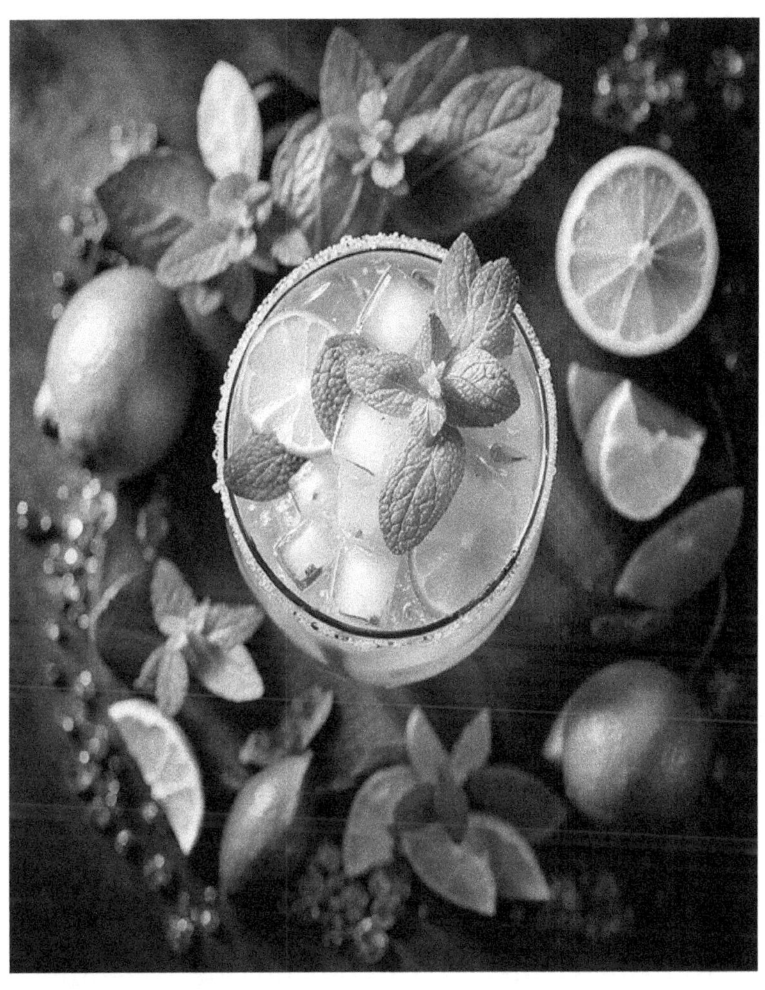

Chapter 6: Meal Planning and Recipes While Fasting

This chapter will walk you through the process of meal planning while fasting, offer you a useful weekly fasting meal calendar, and delve into delicious recipes that promote hormone balance.

Let's explore the realm of perfecting cooking and food planning for maximum health.

Creating and Organizing Meals While Fasting

The key to successfully fasting and reaching your health objectives is meal planning. It requires careful planning, nutrient balance, and adaptability to fit your fasting schedule.

Principles for Planning Meals Well While Fasting

1. Knowing Your Fasting Window:

Determine how long your fasts will last. Understanding your calendar aids in organizing your meals, regardless of whether you want to follow extended fasts or intermittent fasting with a daily eating window.

2. Balancing Macronutrients:

Create meal plans that incorporate a variety of carbohydrates, healthy fats, and proteins. This equilibrium facilitates prolonged energy expenditure and aids in controlling appetite during fasting.

3. Including Nutrient-Dense Foods:

Give whole, nutrient-dense foods top priority. Essential vitamins and minerals are found in fruits, vegetables, lean meats, and whole grains, which promote general health.

4. Variety and Flavor:

To keep things interesting, make sure your

meals are varied. Try varying the herbs, spices, and cooking techniques to enhance taste without sacrificing nutritional content.

5. Meal Preparation:

Take into account meal preparation and bulk cooking. Meal preparation at busy times can be streamlined by having pre-prepared ingredients like cooked grains, roasted veggies, or grilled poultry.

6. Hydration Integration:

Make sure to factor in water while arranging your meals. You can add water, herbal teas, or infused water with fruit and herb slices to your fasting regimen.

7. Adaptability:

Create food plans that are flexible. You may maintain your fasting goals without feeling constrained if you have flexible options because life can be unpredictable.

Quick and Delightful: Hormone Balancing Recipes

Making delectable meals that adhere to fasting guidelines doesn't have to be difficult. Let's look at a few quick and tasty meals that promote hormone balance:

Recipe 1: Roasted Vegetable and Quinoa Salad

Ingredients:

- Quinoa,

-Mixed veggies (zucchini, bell peppers, and cherry tomatoes)

- Olive oil

- Lemon juice

- Fresh herbs, such basil and parsley

- Salt and pepper(add to taste).

Preparation:

1. Prepare the quinoa per the directions on the package.

2. Combine salt, pepper, and olive oil with the chopped veggies. Roast in the oven until soft.

3. Combine roasted veggies and cooked quinoa.

4. Sprinkle fresh herbs over top and drizzle with lemon juice and olive oil.

Recipe 2: Avocado Salsa with Grilled Salmon

Ingredients:

- Avocado,

- Red onion,

- Cilantro,

- Lime juice

- Salmon filets.

- Pepper and salt

Preparation:

1. Cook the salmon filets on the grill until they are thoroughly done.

2. Finely chop the cilantro and red onion, then dice the avocado.

3. To make salsa, combine avocado, cilantro, red onion, and lime juice.

4. Serve avocado salsa over cooked fish.

Recipe 3: Bowl of Stir-fried Chickpeas

Ingredients:

- Cooked or canned chickpeas

- Broccoli, bell peppers, and carrots (are among the mixcd vegetables stir-fried in soy sauce).

- Garlic

- Ginger

- Sesame oil

- Caramel rice

Preparation:

1. Heat sesame oil and sauté the ginger and garlic.

2. Stir-fry the mixed veggies until they become crisp-tender.

3. Stir in the soy sauce and chickpeas, and heat thoroughly.

4. Accompany with cooked brown rice.

Your Weekly Meal Plan for Fasting

Let's now combine everything into a useful weekly fasting food schedule. A variety of recipes and fasting-friendly dinners are included in this sample:

Breakfast: Almond milk and berries with overnight oats.

Lunch: Quinoa salad with roasted vegetables.

Supper: Avocado Salsa paired with Grilled Salmon.

Breakfast: sliced bananas and Greek yogurt with honey.

Lunch: Bowl of stir-fried lentils.

Dinner: Baked chicken breast served with sweet potato wedges for dinner.

On Wednesday:

On Wednesday:

Breakfast: Avocado and whole-grain bread.

Lunch: Mixed greens on the side, along with lentil soup.

Dinner: Grilled shrimp and zucchini noodles with tomato sauce.

Thursday

Breakfast: Omelet of spinach and feta.

Lunch: Wrapped vegetables and turkey.

Supper: Bell peppers filled with quinoa.

Friday

Breakfast: A protein powder, banana, and spinach smoothie.

Lunch: Brown rice bowl with salsa, corn, and black beans for lunch.

Dinner: Stir-fried Teriyaki chicken with brown rice and broccoli.

Breakfast: Chia seed pudding with mango for breakfast.

Lunch: lettuce wraps with tuna salad.

Supper: Quinoa and curry made with eggplant and beans.

Breakfast: Whole Grain pancakes topped with berries for breakfast.

Lunch: Grilled chicken and caprese salad.

Dinner: Baked cod with asparagus for dinner.

You are welcome to modify this calendar to fit your fasting schedule, food requirements, and preferences. The secret is to strike a balance that suits you, including a range of nutrient-dense meals and delectable recipes that will help you make fasting a fun and sustainable part of your life.

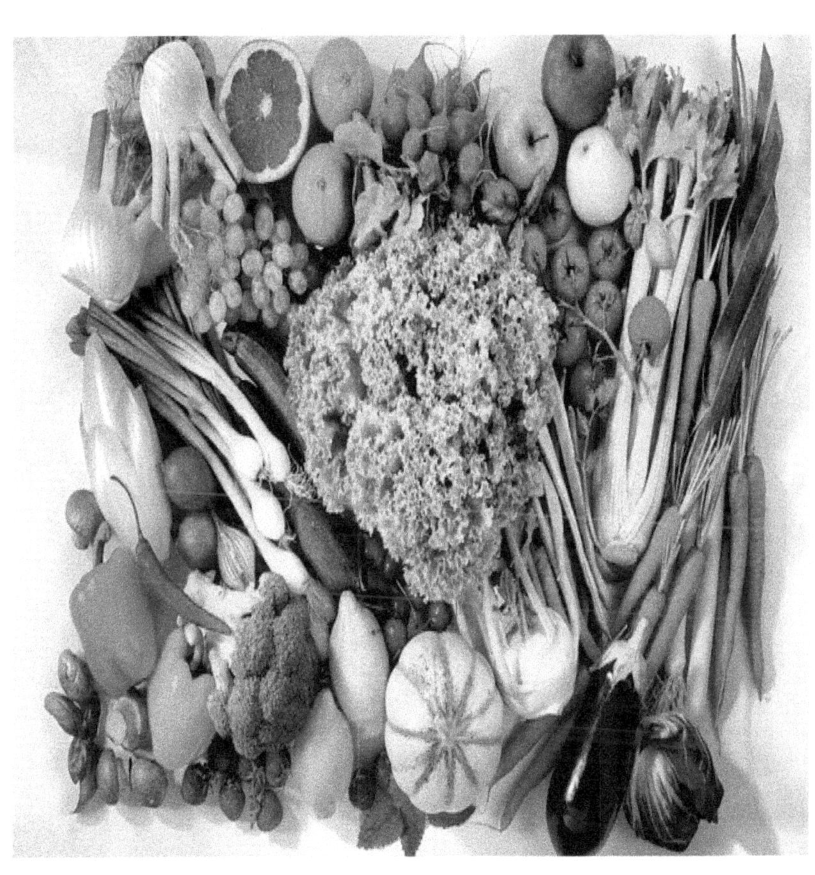

Chapter 7:Integrating Fitness and Lifestyle During Fasting

This chapter will cover the importance of exercise, lifestyle modifications for overall health, and how to combine fasting with fitness in a way that maximizes advantages. Let's explore mobility, modifying our lifestyles, and the benefits of combining fasting with fitness.

The Function of Exercise During Fasting

Exercise is important for maintaining general health and supporting your fasting journey; it's not just about working up a sweat. Let's simplify the function of exercise as follows:

Comprehending the Advantages

1. Caloric Expenditure:

Burning calories through exercise contributes to the caloric balance that is essential for managing weight. It raises energy expenditure, which is a benefit of fasting.

2. Metabolic Boost:

Frequent exercise increases metabolism. This improves your body's ability to use energy, which is consistent with fasting's beneficial effects on metabolism.

3. Muscle Development and Preservation:

Resistance exercise, like lifting weights, promotes the development and preservation of muscle. This is essential during a fast to guarantee that fat, not muscle, is burned off when losing weight.

4. Enhanced Insulin Sensitivity:

Exercise improves insulin sensitivity, which is important for maintaining hormonal equilibrium. This works in concert with fasting to enhance blood sugar regulation.

5. Mood and Well-Being: Endorphins, or "feel-good" hormones, are released when you exercise. This promotes general mental health in addition to helping one maintain an optimistic outlook throughout fasting.

Workout Routines to Try

1. Select Activities You Enjoy:

Pick things that make you happy, such as dancing, weightlifting, walking, or running. Exercise that you enjoy doing has a higher chance of becoming a regular part of your schedule.

2. Start Gradually:

Give your body time to adjust if you're new to exercising. Start with exercises appropriate for your current level of fitness and build up to more strenuous ones.

3. Combine Cardio and Strength Training:

Combine strength training with aerobic exercises (such as cycling or walking). This combo offers a comprehensive approach to fitness.

4. Be Consistent:

Maintaining consistency is essential. Instead of doing short bursts of intensive activity, aim for consistent, sustainable exercise. This fits in nicely with the methodical, step-by-step technique of fasting.

5. Listen to Your Body:

Observe how your body reacts to physical activity. If you feel pain or discomfort, adjust your regimen and get advice from a fitness expert as needed.

Modifications to Lifestyle for Comprehensive Health

In addition to physical activity, modifying

one's lifestyle is essential for attaining overall wellbeing. Let's examine some easy changes that support a better way of living:

Sleep Prioritization:

Enough sleep is necessary for hormone balance and general wellness. Try to get 7-9 hours sleep each night. Create a relaxing sleeping environment and establish a nighttime ritual.

Reduction of Stress:

Hormones might be adversely affected by prolonged stress. Include stress-relieving techniques like deep breathing, meditation, or soothing hobbies.

Hydration Practices:

Drink plenty of water throughout the day. In addition to sustaining biological processes, water can assist control hunger when fasting.

Nutrient-Rich food:

Make sure your food is well-balanced and

high in nutrients. Whole foods supply the vitamins and minerals required for good health.

Social Links:

Foster relationships with others. Social contacts, such as spending time with friends and family or taking part in group activities, are important for emotional health.

Thoughtful Eating:

Make thoughtful food choices. Take note of what you eat, enjoy every meal, and pay attention to your body's signals of hunger and fullness.

Regular Medical Check-ups:

Make an appointment for routine medical examinations with medical specialists to keep an eye on your general health and handle any problems.

Digital Detox:

Take intervals from using screens. Even

short-term digital detoxes can improve mental wellness.

Recreation and Hobbies:

Take part in the things you enjoy. Recreation and hobbies offer a change of pace and support a balanced way of living.

Combining Exercise and Fasting for Optimal Results

The advantages of both fasting and exercise can be increased when they work together. Here's how to easily incorporate them:

Timing Your exercises:

To ensure you have the energy you need for exercise and to speed up recuperation, think about planning your exercises for when you eat.

Hydration During Exercise:

Drink plenty of water, particularly if you're

working out while fasting. Drinks high in electrolytes or water can help with performance.

Post-Workout Nutrition:

To enhance muscle repair and replenish energy stores after workouts, give priority to nutrient-dense meals.

Adapt Exercise Intensity:

During fasting, observe how your body reacts to exercise. Adapting the intensity or timing to your own mood may be necessary.

Diversify Your Workouts:

Combine various exercise styles. heart rate,Exercises for flexibility and strength build general fitness.

Recovery and Rest:

Allocate appropriate days for recuperation and rest. This is essential for general health and muscle recovery, particularly in conjunction with fasting.

Set Realistic Goals:

Make sure your fitness objectives are in line with your fasting schedule. Long-term success is enhanced and sustained by gradual advancement.

Mind-Body Connection:

Encourage a robust mental-physical bond. This entails connecting with your body's signals and requirements while fasting and exercising mindfully.

Celebrate Progress:

Honor accomplishments and advancements. As you stick to your combined fasting and exercise regimen, acknowledge the improvements in your health and fitness.

To sum up, the combination of fasting and exercise produces a potent synergy that leads to comprehensive well-being. Through comprehension of the function of exercise, modification of lifestyle, and synchronization of workouts with fasting, one can set out on a path that advances mental and physical wellness as well as long-term lifestyle choices. Always remember that creating a balanced and meaningful trip is more important than focusing only on the final goal.

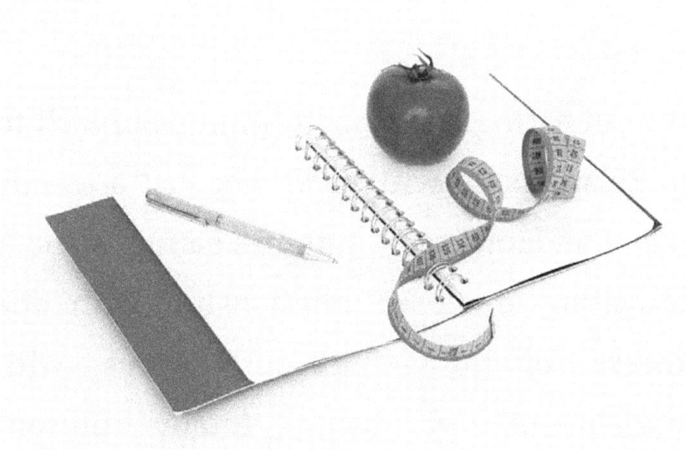

Chapter 8: Mindful Consumption Practices

We will examine how to negotiate fast food mindfully, delve into the art of mindful eating, and discuss typical obstacles to integrating mindfulness into our eating patterns in this chapter. Let's explore straightforward yet deep mindful eating techniques.

Mindful Eating Techniques

Mindful eating is a transforming approach to our relationship with food, not just a trendy term. Fundamentally, mindful eating is about cultivating a closer relationship with the process of providing our bodies with nourishment by being totally present throughout meals. This is a summary of mindful eating techniques:

1. Present Moment Awareness:

Mindful eating asks us to engage with our food in the present. It encourages us to savor each bite and involve all of our senses in the dining experience rather than racing through meals or eating automatically.

2. Paying Attention to Your Body: This exercise helps us become more aware of our bodies' signals of hunger and fullness. We can discern between genuine bodily hunger and emotional or habitual cravings by paying attention to our bodies.

3. Appreciation for Food:

Eating mindfully encourages us to feel thankful for the food we eat. It enhances our appreciation of the tastes, textures, and colors of every meal, fostering a closer bond with the food that is being served.

4. Removing Distractions:

Make a designated area for dining, turn off the TV, and put the phone away. Distractions must be removed in order for us to enjoy our meals and concentrate on the act of eating.

5. Snacking and Feeling Texture:

Eating is made more enjoyable by paying attention to the way food is chewed and feels. Additionally, because the body can metabolize food more effectively, it facilitates healthier digestion.

Recommended Practices for Mindful Eating

1. Slow Down:

Enjoy your food slowly. Between mouthfuls, put down your utensils, chew gently, and give yourself time to really appreciate the tastes.

2. Activate Your Senses:

Take note of the flavors, textures, and colors of your food. Your dining experience is enhanced when you use all of your senses.

3. Express thankfulness:

Give some thought to your thankfulness for the food that is in front of you before you start eating. This easy exercise might change the way you think about food.

4. Pay Attention to Hunger Cues: Before grabbing a snack, check in with your body to see if you're actually hungry. Similarly, notice when you're comfortably satisfied.

5. Mindful Portion Management:

Recognize the sizes of portions. It can be easier to naturally limit quantities and avoid overindulging if you use smaller dishes and bowls.

Mindfully Choosing Fast Food

In a society where there are a lot of quick fast meal options, mindful eating may change everything. Here's how to approach fast food with awareness:

Make a Wise Choice

Select the healthiest options available. Nowadays, a lot of fast-food restaurants provide salads, grilled foods, or portion sizes that are in line with mindful eating.

Savor Every Bite

Try to relish every bite, even in this hectic situation. Chew carefully, and give yourself time to fully appreciate each bite by taking sips between them.

Be Aware of Portion Sizes

Fast food portions are frequently bigger than what our bodies require. Try splitting a meal or putting some food away for later in order to prevent over indulging

Sip water along with your quick food meal. This not only aids in maintaining hydration but also has the potential to promote fullness and curb overindulgence.

Thoughtful Side Selections Consider your selections. Instead of always selecting fries or other high-calorie sides, go for side salads, fruit cups, or other healthy options.

Mindful Eating: Overcoming Common Challenges

Although mindful eating has the potential to change our relationship with food, there are drawbacks. Let's discuss typical obstacles and look at solutions:

1. Time Restrictions

Remedy: Set aside a specific period of time, even if it's only a few minutes, for meals.

Establish a relaxing atmosphere so that you may savor your meal even on hectic days.

2: Emotional Consumption

Remedy: Work on recognizing the feelings that lead to eating. Seek out different coping strategies like writing in a journal, going for a stroll, or speaking with a friend.

3: Outside Distractions

Remedy: Avoid distractions during meals by turning off electronics, TV, and other gadgets. Establish a quiet area where you may concentrate only on your meal.

4: Social Influence

Remedy: Tell your loved ones about your resolve to eat mindfully. Promote a welcoming atmosphere that honors eating with awareness.

5: Unknown Settings

Remedy: Take a moment to calm yourself and breathe when eating in unfamiliar or hectic settings. Try to eat gently and pay attention to what you are eating.

6: Routine Consumption Patterns

Remedy: Make minor adjustments to break bad eating habits. Try attentively attempting new foods or using your non-dominant hand as you eat.

To sum up, mindful eating is an effective technique that changes our connection with food and goes beyond simply eating. We may create a pleasant and durable eating habit by mastering the practice of mindful eating, making thoughtful decisions when it comes to fast food, and overcoming typical obstacles. Never forget that every mindful mouthful is a chance to fuel your body and

mind while also appreciating the richness of
the current moment.

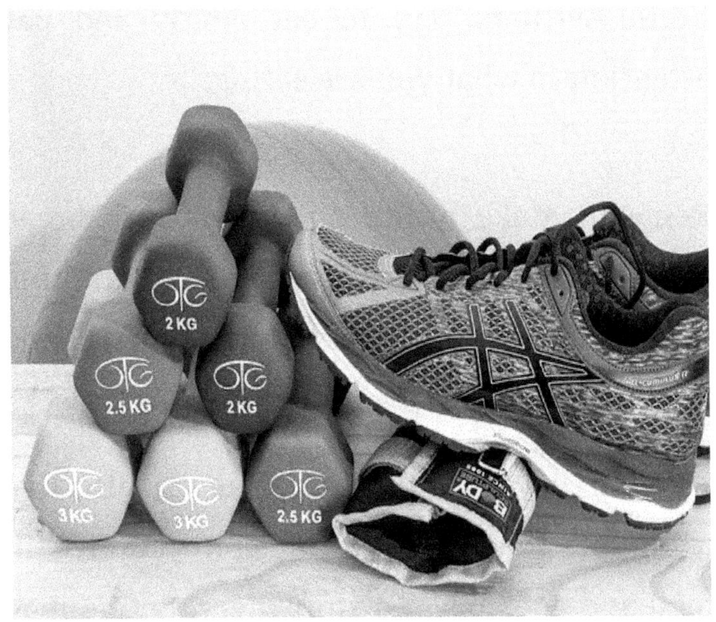

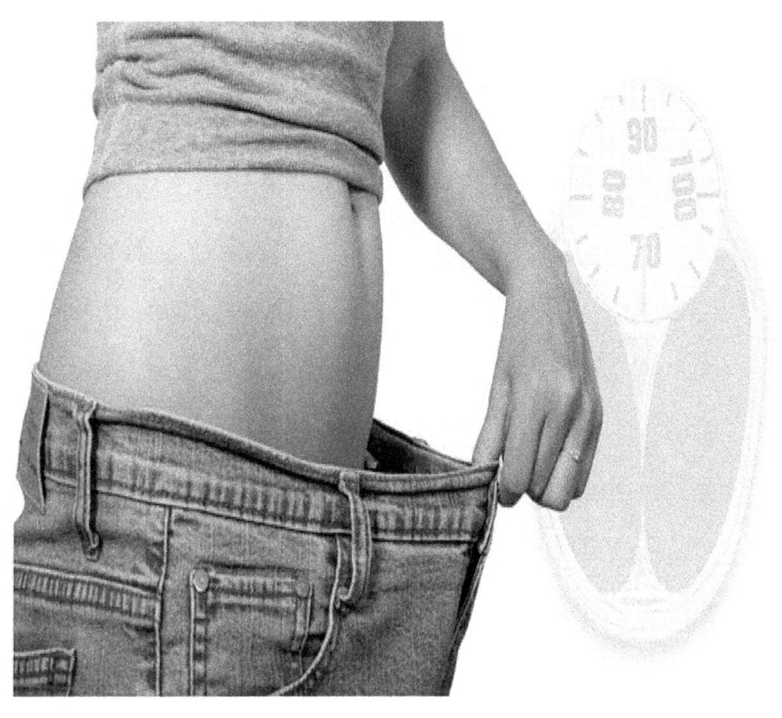

Chapter 9: Uncovering Myths and False claims

Making the difference between reality and fantasy is essential when seeking a healthier lifestyle. The purpose of this chapter is to dispel popular myths about fast food, fasting, and general health. By dispelling misconceptions and illuminating the facts, we enable ourselves to make wise choices for a better future.

Uncovering Myths About Fast Food

Fast food is frequently associated with a negative meaning, such as being fundamentally unhealthy. But it's important to realize that not all fast food is made equally. Making informed decisions is more important than criticizing an entire group.

Myth 1: There Is No Healthy Fast Food

Reality: A lot of restaurants now provide healthier selections, even though certain fast food options are heavy in calories, sugar, and saturated fats. Convenience and nutrition are balanced by the growing popularity of grilled chicken, salads, and fruit selections.

Myth 2: Eating fast food makes you fat

Reality: Genetics, lifestyle, and diet are just a few of the many variables that affect obesity, making it a complicated problem. Simply blaming fast food oversimplifies the issue. Retaining a healthy weight is more dependent on moderation and deliberate decisions.

Myth 3: There's Always Faster Food

Reality: With a little preparation and basic recipes, cooking wholesome meals at home can be done quickly. Fast food may be more convenient in the short run, but the long-term health risks usually outweigh the benefits.

Dispelling Myths Regarding Fasting

Due to its possible health benefits, fasting has become more and more popular; nonetheless, misconceptions about this practice can exist.

Myth 1: Starving Means Fasting

Truth: A regulated, voluntary fasting period involves giving up eating for a predetermined amount of time. Unlike starving, which is unintentional and can have detrimental effects on health, it is voluntary. Fasting may improve a number of health indicators and encourage metabolic flexibility.

Myth 2: Metabolism Is Slowed Down by Fasting

Reality: A brief drop in metabolic rate during a

fast is possible, but this is a normal reaction to preserve energy. Intermittent fasting has been demonstrated to improve metabolic health and weight management over time.

Myth 3: Everyone Can Fast

The truth is that there isn't a single fasting strategy that works for everyone. Some people might not be a good fit for it, including those who are expecting, have specific medical issues, or have a history of eating disorders. It is essential to speak with a healthcare provider before beginning any fasting program.

Understanding Reality to Become a Healthier You

Finding evidence-based facts and cutting through the noise are essential steps in the pursuit of a better lifestyle.

Fact 1: The Key Is Moderation

Achieving equilibrium is crucial. It's acceptable to indulge in fast food indulgences once in a while as long as they're included in a balanced diet. Instead of going completely away, aim for moderation.

Fact 2: Customization Is Important

One person's solution might not be another's. The best diet and fasting strategy vary greatly on a variety of factors, including genetics, lifestyle, and personal preferences. It's important to try several things and see what suits you the best.

Making educated decisions is facilitated by knowledge of the science underlying fasting and the nutritional makeup of fast food. A healthier lifestyle is facilitated by reading labels, paying attention to portion amounts, and maintaining knowledge.

To sum up, debunking misconceptions about fast food and fasting is crucial to helping us make wise decisions regarding our health. The cornerstone of a sustainable and healthy lifestyle is adopting a balanced strategy that takes into account the individuality of health needs and incorporates a range of meals. Personalized decisions, moderation, and education open the door to a path towards wellbeing.

Conclusion

Now that we've completed the "Fast Your Way Out" journey, it's time to take stock of our progress, think about the first steps toward a better version of ourselves, and envision a future free from hormone imbalance, menstrual health issues, and weight gain.

Considering Your Quick Your Journey Out

Your quest for information and dedication to learning about the realm of fasting marked the beginning of your adventure. You've come across myths, overcome obstacles, and seen the transformational potential of deliberate decisions along the journey.

Consider improvements that have been accomplished. No matter how tiny the victory may be, acknowledge it and the lessons it taught you. Fasting is a journey of self-discovery and resilience, not merely skipping meals.

Think about how your health, energy, and general well-being have changed. Observe the mental fortitude acquired from self-control and the realization that being healthy is a journey rather than a destination.

Beginning Your Journey to a Healthier You

Now that your health journey has reached a crossroads, it's time to take those vital first steps toward becoming a healthier version of yourself.

Step 1:Expand on Your Knowledge

The information acquired from the "Fast Your Way Out" adventure is an effective instrument. Recognize the significance of mindful eating, the value of being hydrated, and the fundamentals of balanced nutrition. Use this basis to guide your decision-making.

Step 2: Create Long-Term Habits

Add durable behaviors to your routine instead of depending just on fasting. Make sure you get enough sleep, emphasize regular physical activity, and maintain a varied, nutrient-rich diet. These behaviors are essential to long-term health.

Step 3: Pay Attention to Your Body

Your body expresses what it needs and how it feels. Keep an eye on your energy levels, hunger cues, and the feelings that come with eating different foods. Being aware of this enables you to modify your lifestyle to suit the specific needs of your body.

Welcome to a Future of Menstrual Health, Hormonal Balance, and Weight Control

Imagine a day in the future when menstrual health, hormone balance, and weight control all coexist together.

Hormonal Equilibrium

Although fasting can have a favorable impact on hormonal balance, it's important to know how your body will react to it specifically. Hormones are essential for many body processes, including energy, mood, and metabolism. Maintain hormonal equilibrium by using a holistic strategy that takes lifestyle, stress reduction, and nutrition into account.

Hormonal Wellness

Recognize that fasting may have an impact on menstrual cycles for individuals navigating the challenges of menstrual health. It's critical to place a high priority on general health and, if necessary, seek medical advice. Long-term menstruation health is influenced by an awareness of your body's individual rhythms and the importance of balance.

Weight Management

It takes a diverse approach to manage weight. Consider your general health rather than just the number on the scale. A balanced diet, consistent exercise, and conscientious lifestyle choices are all necessary for sustainable weight control. Accept the differences in your body and its capacity for balance.

In summary, the "Fast Your Way Out" adventure is a starting point for a lifetime commitment to health rather than a finished experience. You give yourself the power to live a happy and full life by taking stock of your path, making conscious efforts to become well, and accepting a future where menstrual health, hormonal balance, and weight management are your main priorities.

Your future well-being is influenced by every wise decision you make today, as health is an ever-changing process. One step at a time, keep going forward on your journey to a healthy you.

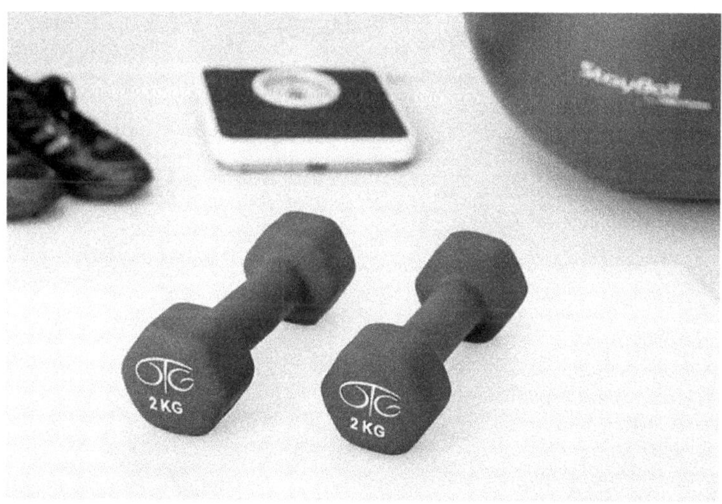